MW01201079

FRENCH FRIES

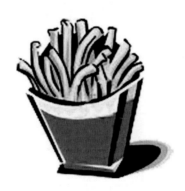

By Lilli Z. Mayerson

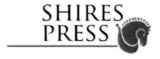

SHIRES
PRESS

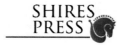

4869 Main Street
P.O. Box 2200
Manchester Center, Vermont 05255
www.northshire.com/printondemand.php

French Fries

Illustrated by Chris Greene
Edited by Karen Dreiblatt

ISBN Number: 978-1-60571-029-7
Library of Congress Number: 2009903552

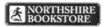

Building Community, One Book at a Time
*This book was printed at the Northshire Bookstore, a family-owned, independent bookstore
in Manchester Center, Vermont, since 1976. We are committed to excellence in bookselling.
The Northshire Bookstore's mission is to serve as a resource for information,
ideas, and entertainment while honoring the needs of customers, staff, and community.*

Printed in the United States of America
using an Espresso Book Machine from On Demand Books

Dedicated to kids who share FRENCH FRIES.

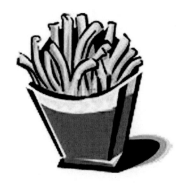

Remember. . .

Every cloud has a silver lining . . .

you just may have to look for it.

Always and everything for my two wise and gentle daughters; for my son who fills my moments with awe and strength; for my parents who first gave me something to write about and who teach me how to be a loving mother for all children; for my in-laws who keep us young; and for my husband who would never eat the last FRENCH FRY *or shrimp in the cocktail.*

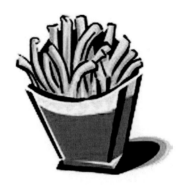

I was having a wonderful life until the day I found out that my little brother, Ben, had *autism*. My mom and I would always bake cookies and go out for nice long morning walks – but we had to stop doing that. My grandma took me out for a walk, but it wasn't the same without my mom.

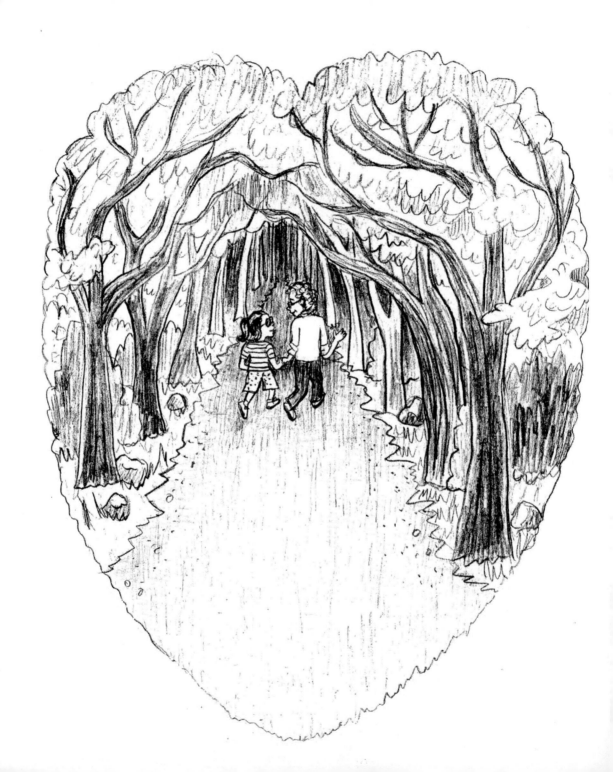

Now let me explain:

Parents and doctors can usually *"diagnose"* autism before a child is three-years old… sometimes they can tell that a baby has autism before it is even one year old.

A child with autism may not be able to use words and they may **make unusual sounds. A child with autism** may also do things like run back and forth and **flap their hands**.

My mother tells me *there are signs* – but I didn't see any of them with my little brother.

My brother was three years old. He didn't say any words, but I always knew what he wanted.

All of a sudden, I *never ever* got to be alone with my mother.

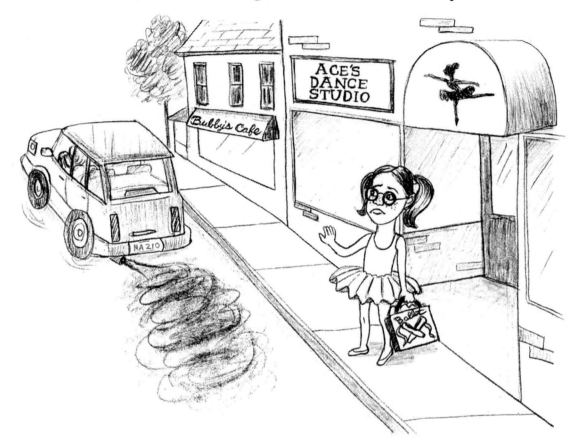

She was **ALWAYS TOO BUSY FOR ME!** For example,
- she could *never ever* go on field trips with my class
- she could *never ever* take me to a play-date
- she could *never ever* go out for ice cream
- she didn't even come inside to watch me at ballet anymore –
  she just dropped me off at the curb…

  AND I WAS ONLY SIX-YEARS-OLD!

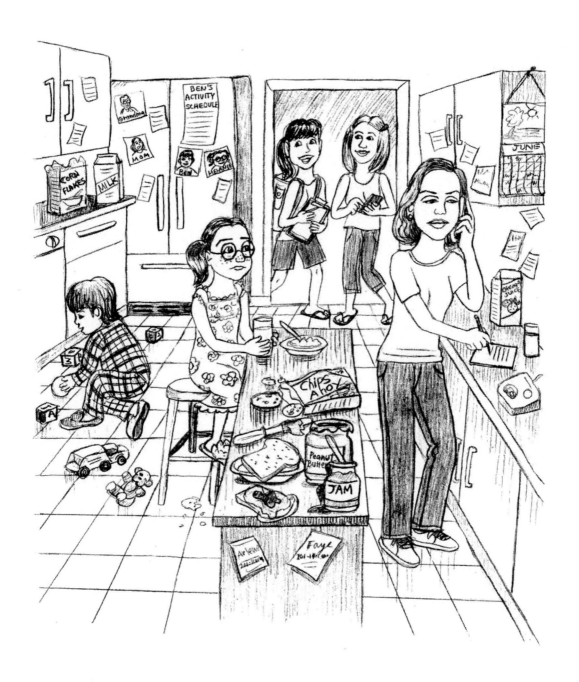

Every day **tutors** (my mother called them *ABA Therapists*) came into our house:

 at breakfast,
 after school,
 during dinner . . .

and **even on weekends!** Sometimes, there were five or six of them over at the same time. My mom called this a "*clinic.*"

Mark was my favorite tutor because he helped Ben learn not to bang on the piano and he once brought me a shampoo with a mermaid on the top. Even though they were all pretty nice, I still **wished they wouldn't come.**

And the *worst thing* was that my mother was **always talking on the phone** –
 ABOUT BEN, of course!

Sometimes, I would watch the therapists teach Ben. I think they made him work too hard because he cried when they were with him. He didn't want to sit in a chair and touch his nose ten times in a row. The snack part was good – when Ben listened, he loved to earn a potato chip.

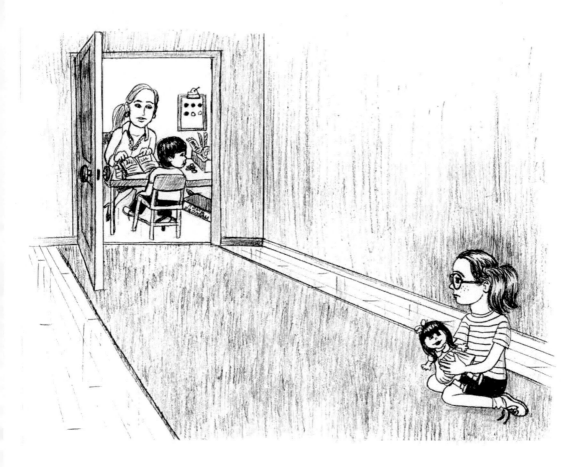

Sometimes I went with my mother and brother to his speech therapy. I think I figured out why Deborah became a *speech therapist* – she talked a lot and loud like we were deaf.

Sometimes Deborah would ask me to come into the room with Ben. Deborah had lots of toys and games. **I was embarrassed** because Ben didn't want to play any of her games; *he just wanted to line-up the same Sesame Street® figures and move them around all by himself.* Deborah let him do it, but she talked to him anyway.

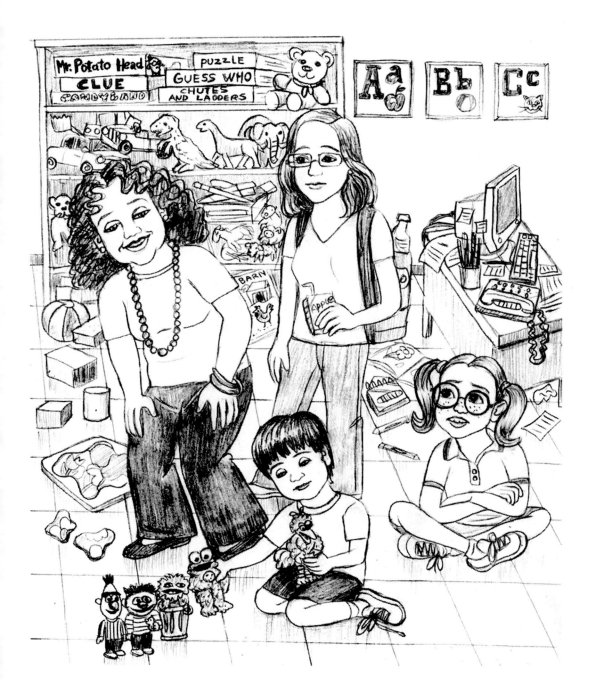

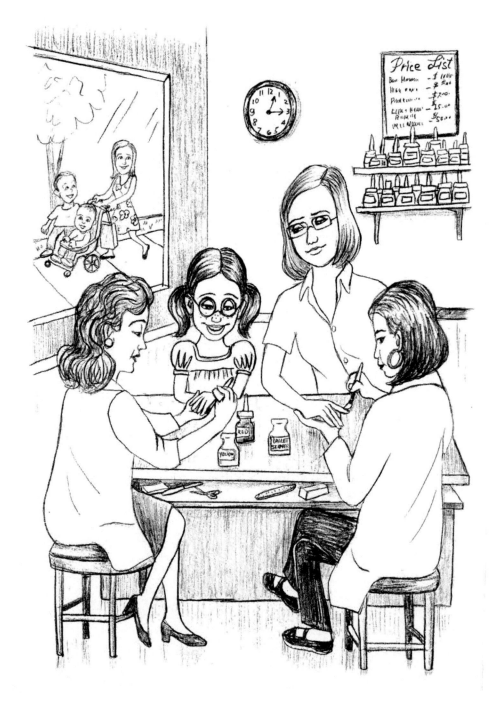

One time, we left Ben with Deborah, and my mom and I went and got manicures. I got bright yellow flowers with a red dot in the middle. My mom got a beigey color called *Ballet Slipper* (I will get that next time).

It was so much fun. We sat next to each other and ate peppermint sucker candies. *I felt so happy* – except that my thumbnail got a big smudge right when I opened the door to leave.

At home, I watched everything like a spy. I saw my mother's worried face and one night I lay in bed and cried into my pillow. When my mother came into my room, I screamed,

"Why do I have to have a brother with autism? I hate him sometimes."

I thought she would be really mad and yell at me, but instead she said softly, *"I know my love. I feel the same way too sometimes."* We cried together and hugged so tight.

I FELT HAPPY AND SAD AT THE SAME TIME.

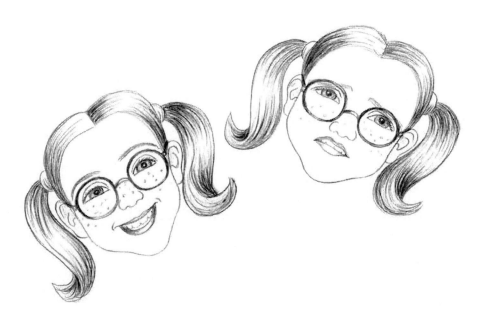

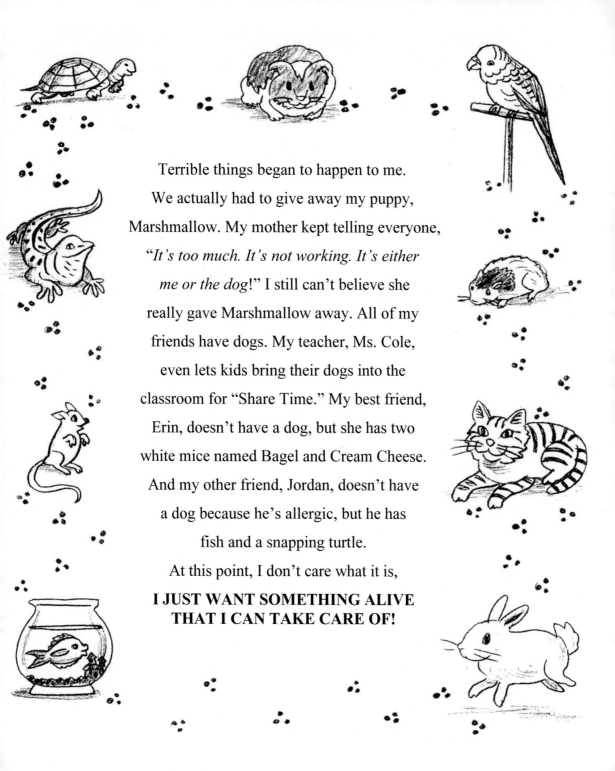

Terrible things began to happen to me. We actually had to give away my puppy, Marshmallow. My mother kept telling everyone, "*It's too much. It's not working. It's either me or the dog!*" I still can't believe she really gave Marshmallow away. All of my friends have dogs. My teacher, Ms. Cole, even lets kids bring their dogs into the classroom for "Share Time." My best friend, Erin, doesn't have a dog, but she has two white mice named Bagel and Cream Cheese. And my other friend, Jordan, doesn't have a dog because he's allergic, but he has fish and a snapping turtle.

At this point, I don't care what it is,

I JUST WANT SOMETHING ALIVE THAT I CAN TAKE CARE OF!

But then one day, the worst thing ever in the entire world happened to me: right after coming home from the doctor for a check-up (it was ok because Dr. Garwood didn't have to give me a shot and she didn't put that stick down my throat), my mother broke the news . . .

She said, "Mel, *sweetheart,* **we have to move!**"

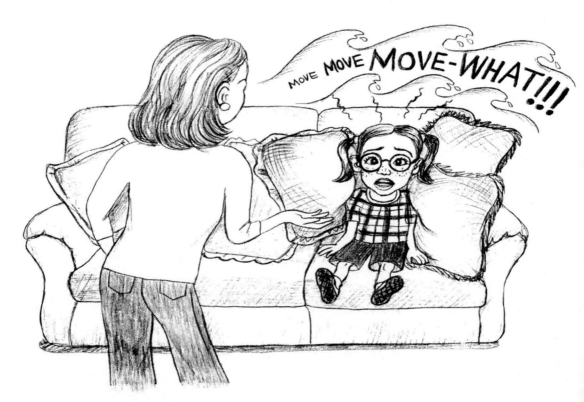

My ears were pounding and my head felt like it was swimming under water. I heard her say, "*Your brother got into a special school in New Jersey . . .*"

Even though my mother's mouth kept moving, I didn't hear anything else.

MOVE!   MOVE AWAY!!

WHAT?   WHEN??   WHERE?
WHY?   WHY??   WHY???

I lived my entire seven-year-old life in this house. This was where I belonged. I couldn't get over it – I didn't have time to get over it because **we moved so fast!**

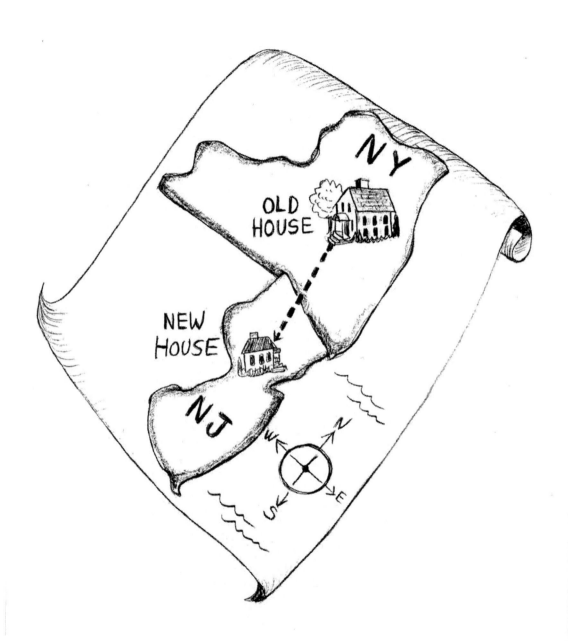

While my mother packed, I went to stay with my Aunt Sue and Uncle Doug, and when I came back it was to a **completely different house in a completely different neighborhood in a completely different state!**

The new house was tiny and dark and it didn't have a front door (or any air conditioners). My room looked like a baby's room. All of my things were in big boxes. I heard my mother say that our furniture was *"in storage"* (whatever that was). The worst part was that the house didn't have a basement, so Ben had to have his therapy in the living room where the TV was.

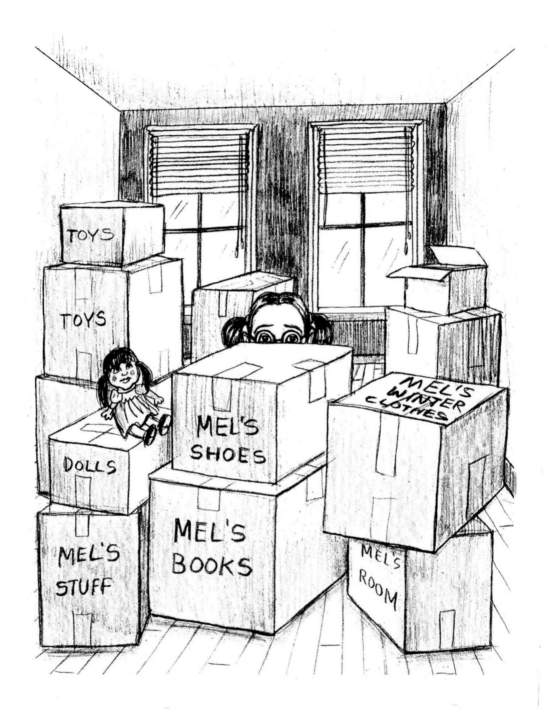

I felt like
there was
nowhere
for me to be.

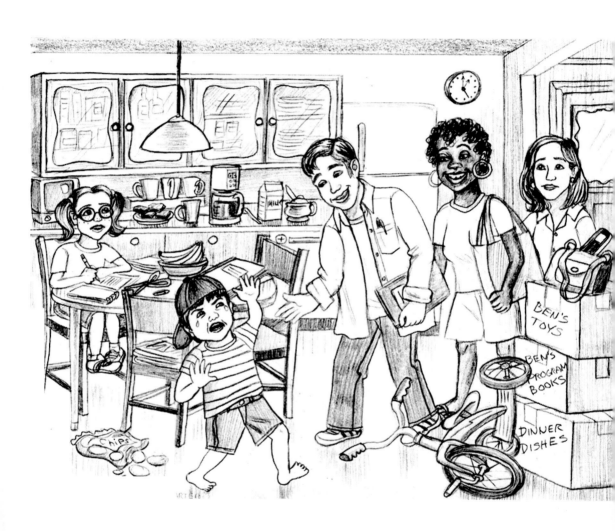

Now all of these strange new therapists (*where did my mother find them?*) came to work with my brother.

"*No Gina*," Ben would **YELL** now.

"*Go away Leslie*," he would SCREAM.

"*Bye-bye Richard*," he would wave as Richard came in the side door.

"*No work Linda*," he would **CRY.**

My brother sure was getting smarter.

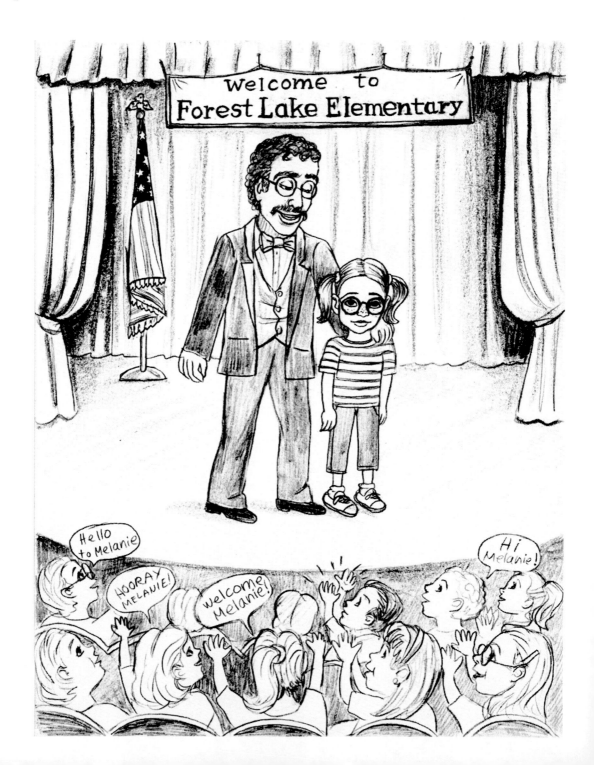

I have to admit that so far my new school is pretty good. On the second day of school, there was an assembly and the principal, Dr. Bartman, called out all the new kids' names. I had to stand up in front of the whole entire school and *everyone clapped* – **JUST FOR ME!** I felt kind of like a celebrity. And then later in the halls, all these kids kept saying hello to me, like they ALWAYS knew me! And my mom is a lunch mom here. She helps serve pizza on Pizza Fridays (and bagels on Bagel Mondays when someone else's mom is sick).

It is really good that Ben goes to school too. The school bus comes right to the side door every morning. The bus driver is really nice. I can tell that he likes driving Ben to school.

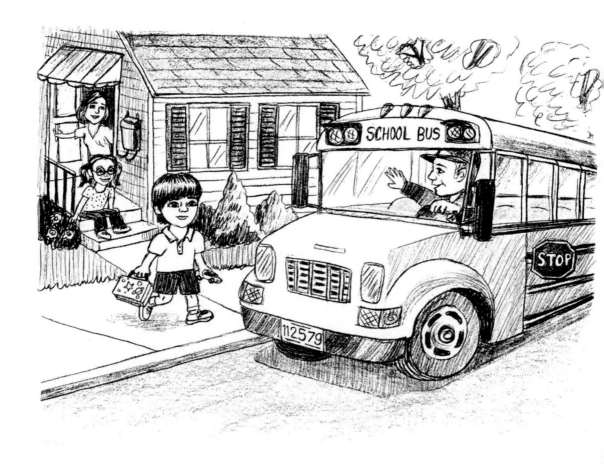

When my mother can take me, I have sleepovers with Erin, my old best friend. I still miss her a lot. I also miss my old bedroom with the puffy painted clouds on my ceiling. And I miss my old backyard with my old special oak tree. I wrote a poem about my special oak tree when I was about four years old.

My Special Oak Tree

Outside is a tree
  that I can see
    that belongs only to me.
      No one else knows
        how happy it grows
          with only the love it receives.

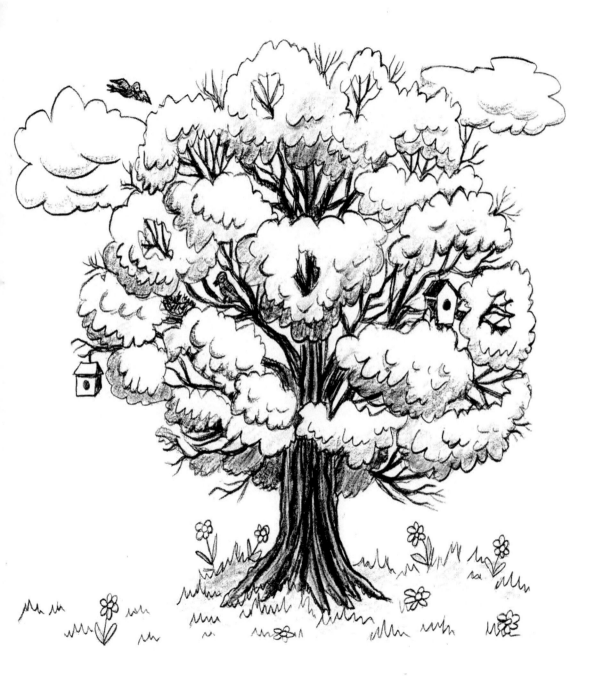

Now my brother is turning into a **HUGE PAIN.** He likes to spill out everyone's drinks on purpose. It is really frustrating. But his most favorite thing to do is to **turn the TV on and off a billion times** – WHILE I am watching it! His therapists try to stop him from doing it. Sometimes they pretend they are leaving the house, but then they hide and catch him "*in the act.*" He doesn't care. He gets hysterical! He won't stop doing it. It is sooooo **annoying!**

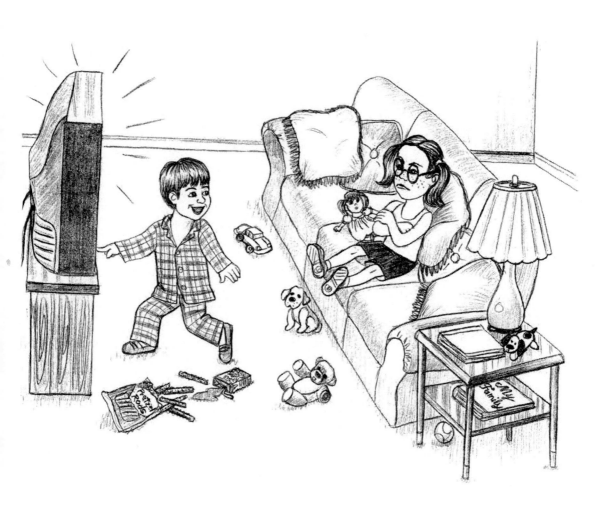

Another hard thing about my brother is that

HE DEFINITELY DOES NOT LIKE TO SHARE . . .

He will **never** let me pick out a game, or give me a red Fruit

Loop®, or let me hold the remote – **he never shares**. . .

especially with FRENCH FRIES –

which just happens to be my very favorite food too!

This FRENCH FRY addiction can be really embarrassing.

Whenever we go out to the diner or even to a fancy restaurant,

if Ben walks by a plate with FRENCH FRIES on it. . . he will just

help himself – just reach out and take one – even if it's from a

complete stranger, or worse – even if it is from a dirty, finished

plate! Of course, this drives my mother (Ms. Antibacterial

Soap) totally crazy and we always end up causing a huge

commotion in the restaurant.

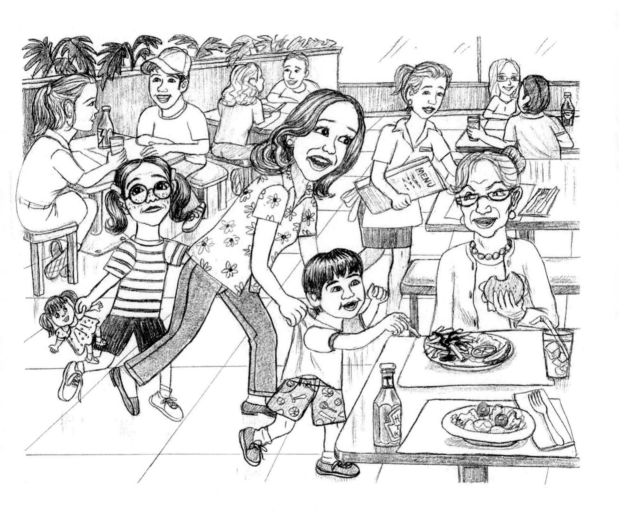

No matter how hard I try to sneak a FRENCH FRY from my brother, he always knows just what I am doing. Sometimes, I plan my attack and wait until his head is completely turned around and then, quick as a flash, I will grab one of his fries.

"*Stop stealing my* FRENCH FRIES," he will scream.

"*Give it back*," he shouts at me. Even if he goes to the bathroom and comes back. . . he always knows the **EXACT** FRENCH FRY count! "*Give them all back*," he demands. His face gets really red and mad – it is soooo **frustrating!**

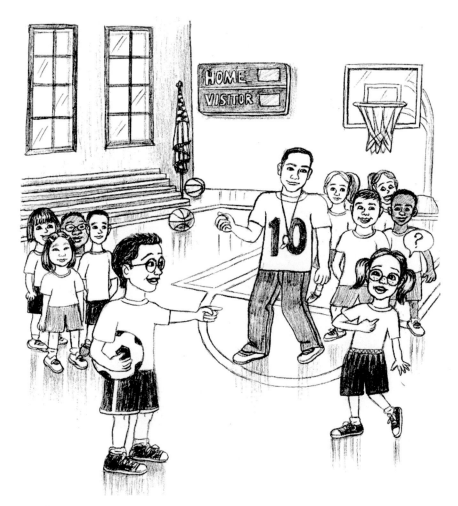

The kids in my new class are OK. There is one boy named
Victor. We have a lot in common: we both wear glasses, we both
have brown hair, and we both have brothers with autism (except
Victor's brother is older than he is). I started to like Victor because
he picked me for his soccer team in gym and I am really terrible in
soccer (in all sports for that matter).

There is one girl I really like the most. Her name is Sandi. She is Chinese and she smiles all the time. She always raises her hand in class and giggles when she gets called on. We had one play-date at my house and the next one will be at her house. Ben likes Sandi, too. He keeps asking me about her.

"Melanie, will Sandi come back to play?"

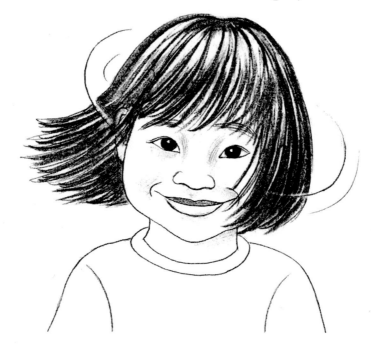

I think Ben likes Sandi because her hair is very shiny and it swishes around her head. Ben likes to touch it. I like Sandi because she doesn't seem to mind. She just smiles.

Sometimes, Ben and I cuddle in his bed at night and he reads to me. He doesn't usually let me read because he likes to do it.

My brother reads better than most of the kids in my class – and I am in the third grade! He loves to say all of the words and he loves when I listen. He gets annoyed when I interrupt him, but that is OK with me because I am very proud that my little brother is such a good reader.

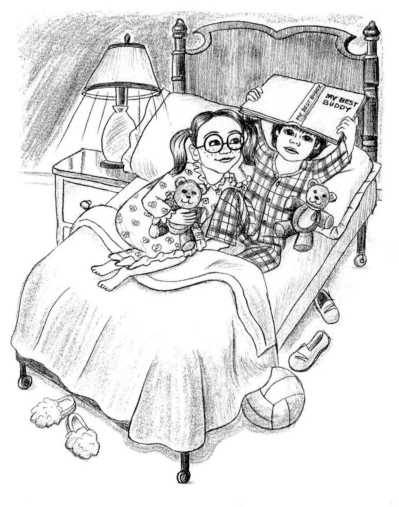

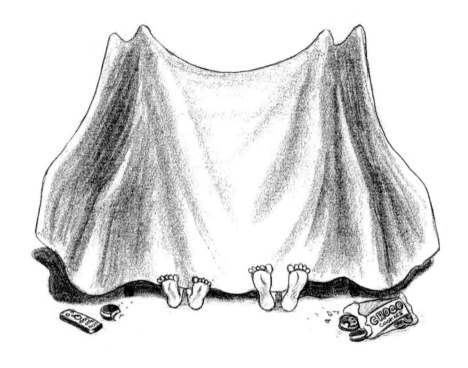

I also love when we make tents out of chairs and blankets in the living room. Even though it gets burning hot inside the tent, he won't let me out.

"STAY IN HERE WITH ME."

The very, very best is when he sometimes says,

"LET'S STAY IN HERE FOREVER, MELANIE."

I love him soooooooooooooooooooo much!

And it is really funny when he yells from upstairs,

**"M - E - L - A - N - I - E . . .
come on - it's time to play tents!"**

My brother is calling my name – how could I refuse that???

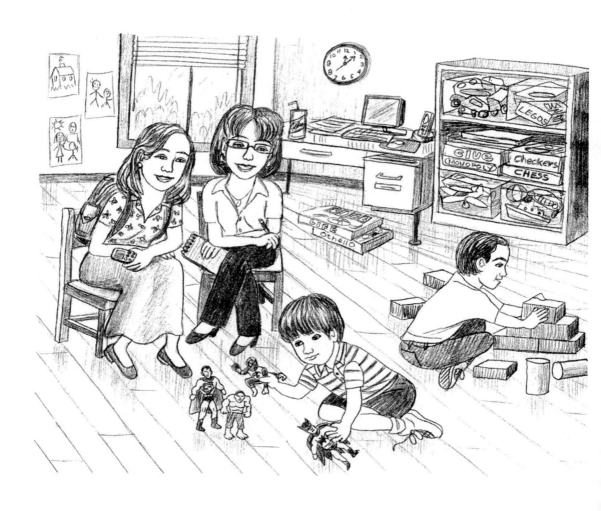

Now Ben has a new speech therapist. Her name is Faye. She is very friendly and asks me a lot of questions about my brother. Faye said that Ben was ready for a *"Social Skills Group"* so now there is another boy, named Ryan, who comes too. Ryan is a little older than Ben and he has *"Asperger's Syndrome."* My mother told me this is a type of autism – she said *Asperger's* is on the "spectrum."

Faye helps Ben and Ryan play together. People with autism can be so different – and so the same. I hear my mother and Faye talk about how **"hard it is for the boys to share."**

I hear them talk about *"eye contact"* and taking turns.

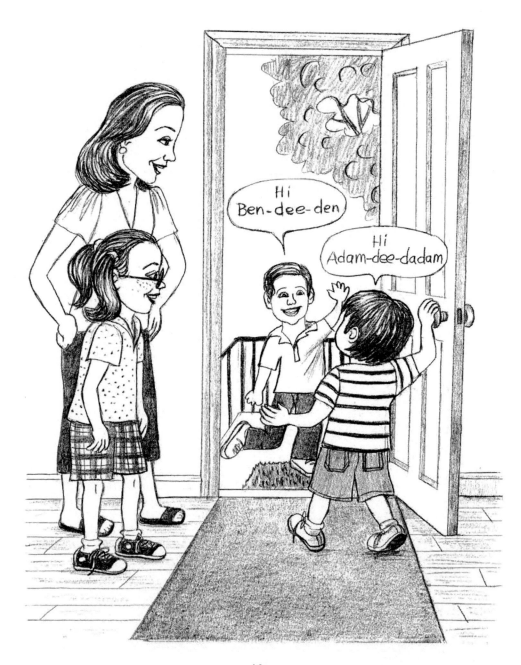

It is very exciting – my brother is really starting to make friends. They come to our house when a therapist is here. It is called "*Peer Modeling*."

"HI, BEN – DEE – DEN," his friend calls.
"HI, ADAM – DEE– DADAM," Ben calls back.

Ben is getting really good at copying what his friends do. Ben and Adam play with blocks and action figures and if Ben is really good – he gets to play video games with his friends.

Sometimes, my mother videotapes Ben playing with a friend and then she shows it to Ben's therapists. I am not sure what they are looking for.

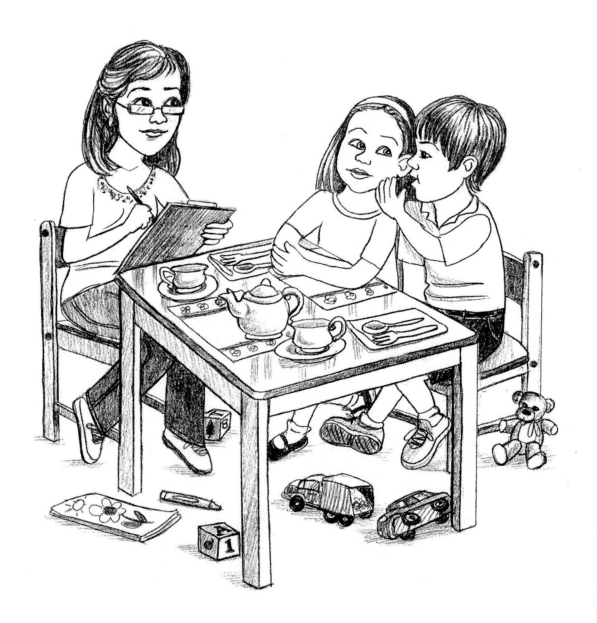

It's great that my mother made a new friend named Judie. Judie's son, Jake, is my exact age. Jake has autism and goes to Ben's school. Judie also has a daughter named Annie. Annie is Ben's age. Annie's face looks like a sweet apple. Annie comes over to play with Ben every Monday. I just wish Ben's therapist would let them do some "boy" things – I don't think my brother really likes to "play house" all the time.

"Annie, lets play computer." Ben says, a little too loudly.

Annie is shy and she quietly responds, *"Not now Ben, maybe later."*

One day, my mother tells me that Jake is going to start coming over on Mondays, too . . . TO PLAY WITH ME! She explains that Jake does not have any friends and that he will bring his own therapist to help him learn to play. This makes me very nervous. I am a skinny, eight-and-a-half-year-old girl – WHAT WOULD I SAY TO A BOY? My mother tells me that Jake is a very good reader just like me and that he knows a lot about Disney characters. She says that Jake is "delicious." Did I ever mention that my mother is weird? (Sometimes she just looks at me and starts to cry – for no reason.)

BIG SURPRISE – I really have fun when Jake comes over! He reminds me of my brother, except that my brother talks a lot more. **When we play, I forget he has autism**.

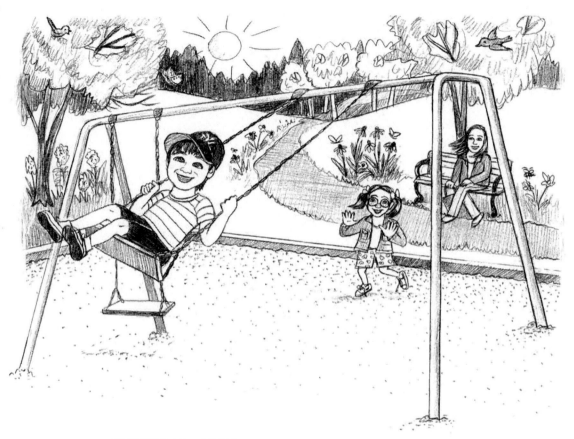

HURRAY! Finally, Ben's therapists don't come on

Sunday anymore! We have a ***FREE*** day so we usually go to a really

cool park. I love to watch my brother on the swings – he is so happy.

My mother and I take turns pushing him – he could stay on the swings

all day long.

Now there is a completely new thing Ben does that drives me crazy. HE WILL NOT GO TO SLEEP! He thinks this is very funny. He comes out of his bedroom about a hundred times every night and he talks really loudly.

"MOM, WHERE ARE YOUUUUUUU?" he yells.

The other night *(it was a school night)*, Ben burst into my bedroom and turned on my light and yelled,

"MEL, I HAVE TO TELL YOU SOMETHING!"

It was almost one o'clock in the morning. My mother got really angry. She was (almost) mean to my brother. She kept saying, *"Not now Ben. Stay in your room Ben. It is the middle of the night! I can never get a second off from you kids!"*

Even though she yelled a lot, my brother kept coming out of his room. I was so tired, I just started to laugh. It was so ridiculous. Then my mother came into my bedroom and I thought for sure she would be mad, but she was laughing too.

"It's too much, too much," she said to me.

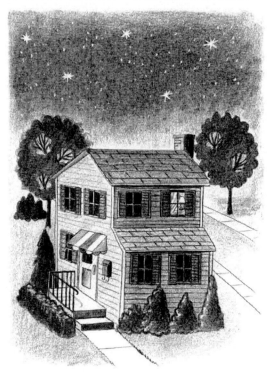

She climbed into my bed and we hugged so tight. I guess after a while, Ben fell asleep too.

I love going out to dinner with my family – it reminds me of "old times." I definitely feel like I am growing up and getting too big for the children's menu because the last time we went out to dinner, even after I ate my whole entire plate of spaghetti (and four pieces of garlic bread), I was still hungry. My mother was eating a salad with strange looking things in it. I looked over at Ben. He was minding his own business, happily eating his cheeseburger deluxe. He was eating very slowly and neatly, as usual.

"Hey, Ben," I said. *"I just finished my whole entire dinner and I am still hungry."* (Believe me - I do not know why I said this!)

"Here, Sis," Ben said. He held his chubby, greasy hand out to me.

"HAVE A FRENCH FRY."

My mother smiled and then she started to cry. I know she is getting happier.

I KNOW I AM HAPPIER TOO!

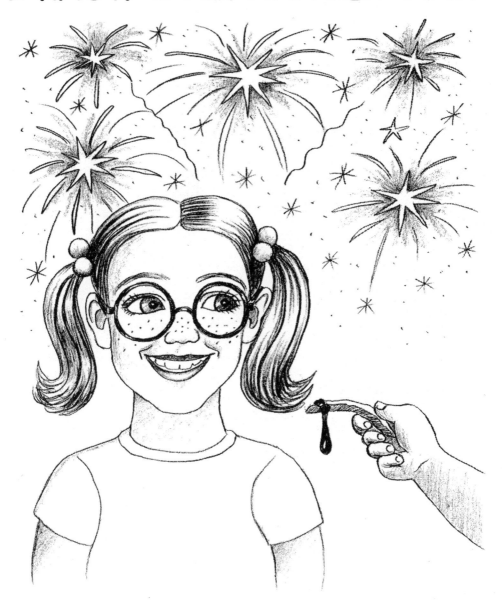

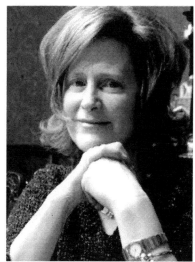

Photo by Matt Mayerson

Lilli Z. Mayerson

Lilli Z. Mayerson has a big old trunk filled with diaries that she has kept ever since she was a little girl. She writes about her feelings and the people that she loves. She has a lot of stories to tell. If you would like to share a story with Lilli, you can contact her at info@lzmayerson.com or visit her website at www.lzmayerson.com.

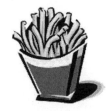